Creative Stoner Journal

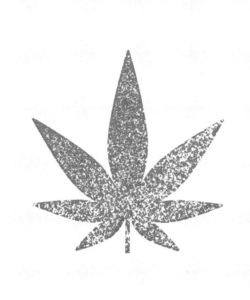

CREATIVE STONER JOURNAL

150 MIND-EXPANDING PROMPTS TO UNLEASH YOUR IMAGINATION WHILE HIGH

OLIVIA ALEXANDER

ROCKRIDGE
PRESS

Copyright © 2022 by Rockridge Press

First Rockridge Press trade paperback edition 2022

Rockridge Press and the Rockridge Press logo are trademarks or registered trademarks of Callisto Media Inc. and/or its affiliates in the United States and other countries and may not be used without written permission.

For general information on our other products and services, please contact our Customer Care Department within the United States at (866) 744-2665, or outside the United States at (510) 253-0500.

Paperback ISBN: 979-8-88608-038-4

Manufactured in the United States of America

Interior and Cover Designer: Chiaka John
Art Producer: Megan Baggott
Editor: Anna Pulley
Production Manager: Martin Worthington

Illustrations © Watercolor fantasy 26/Creative Market, cover and pp. iii, viii, xi, 1, 33, 65, 97, 129; © Brenna Daugherty, pp. vi, viii, ix, x, xii, 1, 2, 5, 6, 9, 10, 13, 14, 17, 18, 21, 22, 25, 26, 29, 30, 32-34, 37, 38, 41, 42, 45, 46, 49, 50, 53, 54, 57, 58, 61, 62, 64-66, 69, 70, 73, 74, 77, 78, 81, 82, 85, 86, 89, 90, 93, 94, 96-98, 101, 102, 105, 106, 109, 110, 113, 114, 117, 118, 121, 122, 125, 126, 128- 130, 133, 134, 137, 138, 141, 142, 145, 146, 149, 150, 152, 154, 157, 158; all other illustrations used under license from iStock; author photo courtesy of Molly Pan Photography.

10 9 8 7 6 5 4 3 2 1 0

This Journal Belongs to:

_____

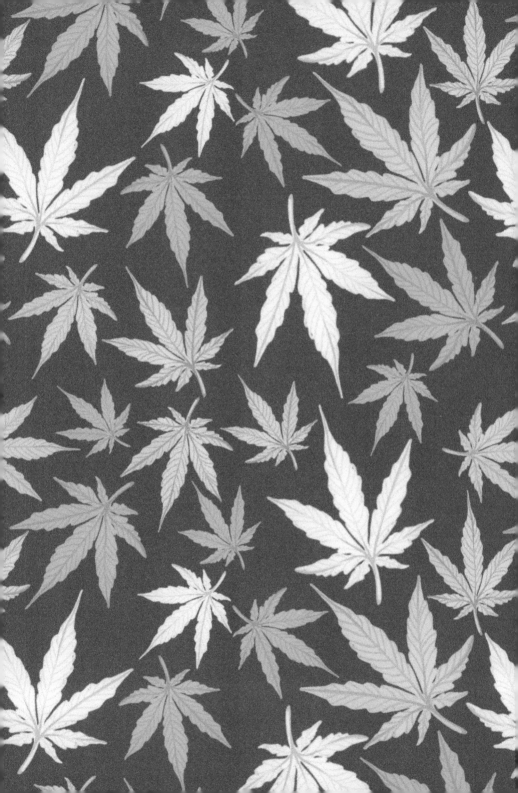

Introduction

Welcome to your *Creative Stoner Journal*! I'm Olivia Alexander, a cannabis advocate and entrepreneur, and I'll be your guide on this journey to unlock the "plant magic" inside of you. I have been consuming cannabis and working in the industry for over sixteen years and am a lifelong creative. I love to use cannabis to unlock my imagination, explore new ideas, and just have fun.

Yes, cannabis is a plant, but it's also a tool to free your mind and uncover the creativity inside of you. The human body's endocannabinoid system, also known as ECS, interacts with cannabinoid molecules from cannabis to heighten the senses and relax the mind, allowing our thoughts and perceptions to change. Using this journal, you're going to explore the creative mindset brought about through cannabis. Think of this book as a journey, and each prompt as a new adventure.

You might be wondering about the scientific reasons for how cannabis increases our creativity. All cannabis science is relatively new, but there is a ton of interesting research, including a number of published studies that show the plant's ability to increase blood flow to the frontal lobe of the brain, where all our creative "outside-the-box" thinking occurs. There's also evidence, as published in *Berkeley Medical Journal*, that cannabis allows your neurons to move more uninhibitedly.

Cannabis is also known as a creative maximizer, because it deactivates certain parts of the brain, including our "judgy brain" (also called the dorsolateral prefrontal cortex), which, when released of constraints and criticism, allows ideas to flow freely. This same part of the brain manages the cognitive control of our emotions, including planning, self-censoring thoughts, and managing our inhibitions. Turning down this part of our brain allows us to daydream, meditate, and explore altered states of consciousness as we focus more easily and let our imagination run wild—thus, the "plant magic" I referred to at the beginning of this introduction.

While all of this sounds very enjoyable, I want to note that this journal is not designed to be used for coping with depression or anxiety, though cannabis can be helpful for those conditions. Instead, this book is simply intended to allow you to explore the creative mindset and free thinking that comes from ingesting cannabis.

If you're new to using cannabis, less is often more. "Start low and go slow" is the best approach for new users. If you're an old pro, you know your tolerance and body best, so just continue to trust yourself. When you're exploring cannabis for creativity, the setting is another important aspect. You could be outside in nature, at your desk, in your backyard, or even at the beach. Wherever you are, just try to limit distractions for best practice.

A little advance preparation before you start writing can also help you focus on your thoughts and not be distracted by the need to grab things. First, you'll want to consider your delivery method when using this journal, whether that be through joints, bowls, edibles, beverages, or vaping. You'll also want to consider the strain and terpene profile of the plant you're consuming. For creativity, I recommend sativa-dominant strains like Jack Herer, Chemdog, Barry White, Jilly Bean, Tangie, or Purple Haze. I love to have a refreshing drink nearby for my dry mouth and a healthy snack in case I get the munchies.

As you move through the prompts, I encourage you to remain as present as possible and welcome new thoughts as they come to you. Let the plant help relax you and connect you to your highest self (pun unintended). This is a judgment-free zone, and we're here to have a good time. It's time to have some fun, so roll up, pop a gummy, or pack a bowl. (Maybe you'll do all three!) The journey begins now.

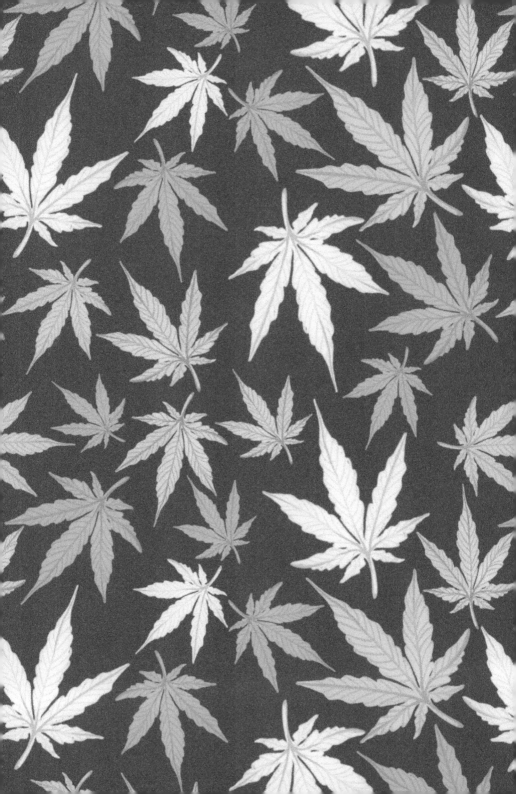

How to Use This Book

his journal includes five themed sections: Outer Space, Nature, Food, The Self, and The Past. In each section are thirty prompts to stimulate your creativity and provide space for you to explore your thoughts. Some will be specifically about cannabis, others won't. There are no rules here, so please explore this journal as you wish. You could explore the prompts chronologically, from start to finish, or skip around the sections, depending on what you're feeling that day. This journal is about you, and there's no wrong way to engage with it. I suggest taking a few deep breaths and letting your high settle before you decide where you want to explore. You may get high and be in a more spacey mood and choose to do a few prompts in each section. You may use a strain that makes you feel more introspective and want to skip right to The Self. You may have time to devote an hour to writing or only have time for a single prompt. This book is available on your time, so choose your own adventure of creative exploration as it works for you.

One thing to keep in mind is the benefit of regular creative practice. The more consistently you are able to come back to this journal and make it a regular practice, the more it will flow, and the more you will get out of it in the way of peace, clarity, confidence, and enjoyment.

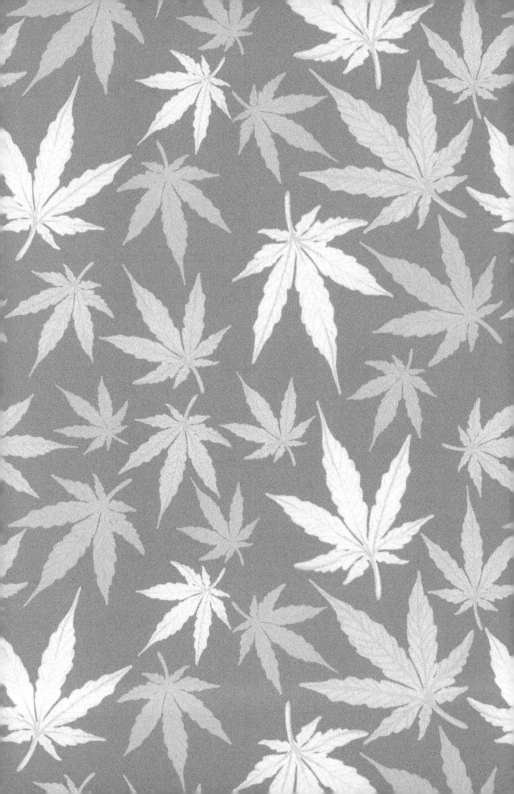

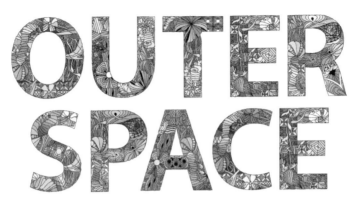

OUTER SPACE

The universe is a vast and never-ending source of curiosity and inspiration. It has captured the interest of creative minds and civilizations for thousands of years. The prompts in this section will put the space in "space cake" by encouraging you to contemplate the greater unknown. If you're looking to pair this section with a strain, I recommend Space Candy, Northern Lights, Cosmic Collision, and Apollo 11, which all brought me far out (in the best way). Now, take a deep breath and give yourself some space to journey out of this world.

You've traveled far into outer space to bring cannabis to a newly discovered extra-terrestrial civilization. In addition, you get to build and oversee this new civilization. What do they look like? Will you set rules or let its inhabitants be free?

Create a short playlist of your favorite space-themed movies to watch next time you're couch-locked.

You just got super stoned. You're zooming around in space, and you meet an alien. You invite them to show you around. Describe this high adventure with your new alien friend.

Invent your own planet. What's its origin story? What's it like?

Is our universe the only one?

You're able to peer just beyond the observable universe. Describe in detail
what you see.

What do stars taste like? Feel like? Sound like?
Use as many of your senses as you can.

You've traveled beyond our solar system and reached another galaxy. You see a supernova (a star explosion) and venture near. How do you feel? Are you scared? Excited? Describe the experience.

You discover a new planet and have been there for a few months, but now you must carry on with your exploration. Leave behind three notes for the next explorer who discovers your planet.

Pluto's not a planet anymore. Write Pluto a short letter.

What does space smell like?

It's been 420 years since you left Earth, and now you're returning home. What has changed? How have you changed?

You've jumped aboard a spaceship and taken control. Where to, Captain?

Saturn's rings have become an edible. When the high hits, you're spit out into a galaxy far away. What happens when you're high and floating in a faraway galaxy?

You've traveled deep into space, tens of thousands of light-years beyond our galaxy, to make a new discovery. What do you find? Describe it in detail in a paragraph to send back to Earth.

"Hotboxing" is the concept of smoking cannabis in a confined area with no ventilation. Well, you get to hotbox the International Space Station with one astronaut. Who do you choose and what happens?

You experience something no one else has: You survive entering a black hole. What is it like, and what do you learn from it?

_____

_____

_____

_____

_____

_____

_____

_____

_____

_____

_____

_____

_____

_____

_____

No astronaut has ever consumed cannabis in space (on record), because too much could go wrong. You get to be the first person to do so. What would your sesh look like?

Why does outer space exist? Why do we?

If untrained humans could move through inter-
stellar space, would you want to float out in
the ether or travel in a spaceship? Why?

"Space rocks" are cannabis-infused Pop Rocks that get you high. You crack open a package and toss back the space rocks. The pop in your mouth and the faint taste of weed hits your tastebuds. Snap, crackle, they pop in your mouth. As the space rocks hit you, time slows and your eyes get higher. You fall into a deep sleep and wake up on a rock in space. Finish this story of your space rock dream-trip.

If you could journey to any planet or galaxy currently known to humankind, what place would you choose, and why?

It's speculated that Mars will potentially be inhabited by humans someday. You get to journey to Mars first, to bury a time capsule. What five things would you put inside your time capsule, and why?

What's one mystery you have always wondered about the universe? Ponder how to solve that mystery.

There are an estimated two trillion galaxies in space. You find a new one. What do you name it, and how did you discover it?

Are we alone in the universe? Or do other lifeforms exist?

You get to send out three messages into space. You don't know who will receive them or where they will land in the galaxy. What messages do you send out to the ether?

_____

_____

_____

_____

_____

_____

_____

_____

_____

_____

_____

_____

_____

_____

_____

_____

You're traveling at high speed through space. Colors are flying everywhere, and you're seeing asteroids, stars, and planets up close and in great detail. Describe what you see.

Think about the way it feels to be weightless, like when you're swimming in a pool. Except now you're floating in space, and there is no such thing as time. Write down the first three thoughts that come to mind.

Venus and Mars are having a conversation about something very important. Create the dialogue of this scene.

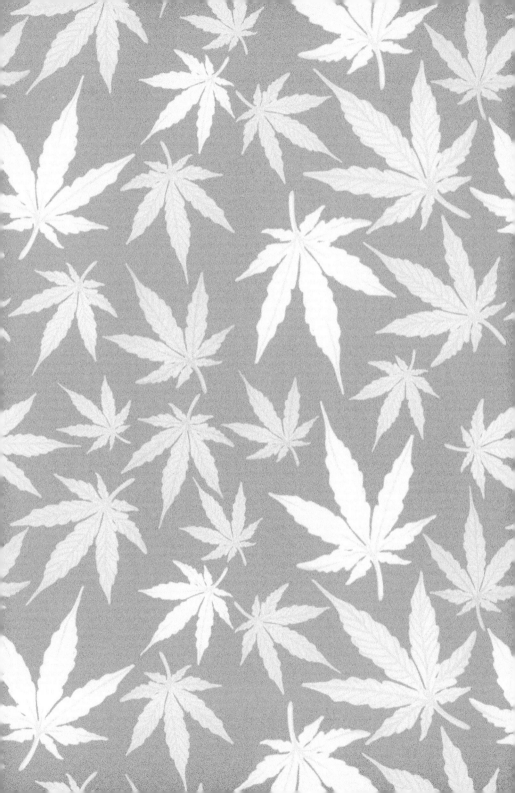

NATURE

Now that you've journeyed through space and the great beyond, I invite you back to Earth to explore the wonders of nature. The cannabis plant is just one example of the endless fascination that is the natural world. The plant itself has grown on Earth for thousands of years and evolved alongside humans. It heightens our senses to help us connect more deeply to the planet. My favorite strains for this section are Blue Dream, Jack Herer, Wedding Cake, Durban Poison, Xeno, and Biskante. I invite you to turn up your senses to take advantage of nature's vast richness. As I write this, I am listening to the sound of rain. Opening my windows, I can smell the ocean air. Ready to join me? Good—let's explore the wonder that is Mother Nature and tap into her never-ending well of creativity.

You are a part of nature and its four elements: fire, air, water, and earth. Which element do you most relate to, and why?

Find a spot to observe nature. You could be in your home and looking through a window at a tree or plant, or sitting on top of a mountain, or deep inside a forest. Spend five minutes mindfully observing your surroundings and write down what you see and experience.

Imagine you're sitting by a campfire on the beach. The fire crackles and pops, and the smell of smoke fills the air. You can hear the waves crashing along the shore. The stars are scattered throughout the sky on this perfectly clear night. What happens next?

You decide you're going off the grid. You can pick anywhere in the world to set up your new home. Where would you go, and what ten items would you bring?

If you could ask Earth three questions, what would they be?

You climb up into a beautiful tree and sit on its branches. You kick off a conversation with the tree. What do you say, and what does it say back?

You're in the middle of a vast field of flowers known as a "super bloom." It's endless and majestic. Just when you think it can't get any more beautiful, hundreds of butterflies flutter in. Write down how you feel about the wonder of this moment.

Flowers have such unique fragrances, just like cannabis. Describe in detail the scent of a cannabis flower. (All the better if you can smell it while you write.)

Cannabis is plant magic, but for this prompt let's pretend that by smoking it you can travel anywhere on Earth for your high. Where do you wish this high would take you and what happens?

A hummingbird hovers right next to you for a few brief moments. It's communing with you. What does it have to tell you?

Let's put the "high" in hiking. Pick your strain and then plan an epic hike. It could be a snow hike with hot chocolate, a coastal hike with scenic views, or a forest hike in Redwood National Park or the White Mountains.

Complete this prompt: When I am alone in
nature, I feel . . .

You're out for a day hike with some cannabis-infused trail mix. It's a micro dose for the perfect hike high. You have a few handfuls and begin to feel the effects, then you come to a majestic waterfall. Its over 100-feet high and crashing into a pool of water. You dive in and have a stoned swim. Describe the waterfall and the way the water feels on your skin.

There are so many incredible beaches in the world. Wide, flat beaches and short, rocky beaches. Black sand beaches, as well as pink-, orange-, and even green-sand beaches. Describe your ideal beach.

You are sitting in a clear kayak on a crystalline blue lake. You can see the bottom as clearly as in a swimming pool. You spot huge boulders under the water and decide to put on a snorkel and goggles to explore further. Describe what you see.

You get to have a national park to yourself for a day—any national park in the entire world. What national park would you pick, and what would you do with the twenty-four hours that it's all yours?

You come across a magical forked path in the woods, which allows you to "do-over" one major life event. What event from your past do you choose and what changes?

You walk into a soft, grassy field. The grass sways in the wind, and you see a hawk flying above you. The hawk guides you to walk down a bend, where you see a big forest. What happens next? Finish the journey of you and your hawk.

You reach the top of a massive and majestic mountain. The view is unlike anything you've ever seen. In only twenty-five words, describe the sights, sounds, and smells.

What is beauty?

I once visited an old tree in Mexico named La Abuela (The Grandmother). She was over 200 years old. She was so large that her trunk was said to be full of wisdom. When we got to the tree, we were told to ask her three questions. What three questions would you ask La Abuela?

In the first prompt of this section (page 34), you chose your favorite element of nature. Today, you are one with that element. How does that element fill you? Where does it take you, and what do you do with this power?

You inhale the best cannabis you have ever smoked. When you exhale, the smoke doesn't dissipate; it becomes clouds. What do your smoke clouds look like? Describe them in detail.

You encounter your animal avatar in nature. What kind of animal is it, and what does it tell you?

You're deep in the rainforest. As you settle into a place to rest, you spy something poking out of the mud. You unearth a box, and inside it is a jar of cannabis joints. On the jar is a note that reads, "Smoke me if found." Do you smoke the joints? What is the reason you do or do not smoke them?

You get one free opportunity to teleport to any spot in the world—the only condition is that the spot must be natural. It could be famous or unknown; near or far. What spot do you teleport to, and why?

You've got the munchies real bad, but you're off the beaten path in the middle of nowhere. Just as you run out of food, a magical tree full of fruit appears. What kind of fruit is it? Describe the way it smells, feels, and tastes as you pick it from the tree and devour it.

You're on the famous Flamingo Beach in Aruba. Flamingos surround you and begin to dance. Make a five-song playlist for dancing with the flamingos.

Think of an imaginary landscape that you would like to explore while high. What are its features? What does it sound like? How do you explore it?

Sound bathing is a meditative practice that involves immersing yourself in sounds. Create your own sound bath in nature, if you can, or by playing some soothing nature sounds at home. Describe the experience and how you felt afterward.

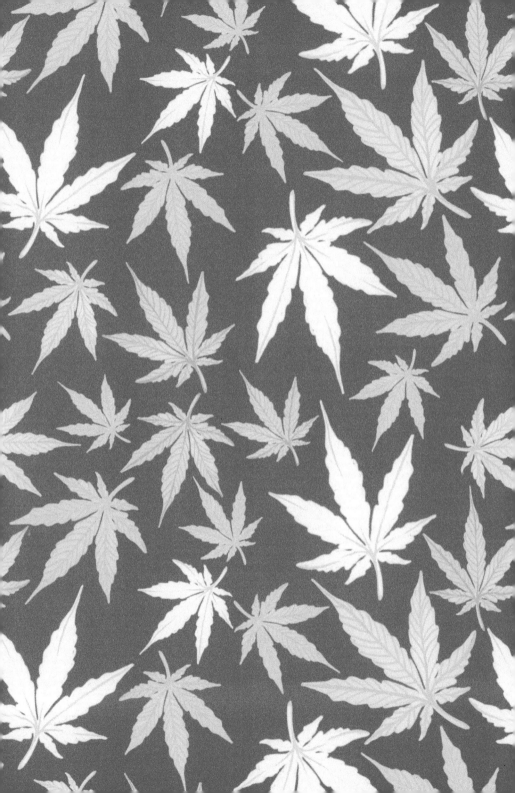

FOOD

Cannabis and food. Was there ever a more iconic duo? Cannabis and food are so powerfully intertwined because of our endocannabinoid system. Yes, most cannabis gives you the munchies and stimulates your appetite, but the endocannabinoid system also rewards you with euphoric brain molecules for eating while high. Your senses are literally heightened, enhancing the pleasure of food even more. In this section, we'll explore cannabis and food for the purpose of creativity. My favorite strains for this section are GSC, Sour Diesel, OG Kush, and Pineapple Kush. Sativa strains often have the ability to suppress the appetite, so lean more toward indica and hybrid strains. Bong appétit!

What's the best thing you've ever tasted or eaten?

Picture your dream munchie-spread. What would it contain? Who would you invite to join you?

You have your own chef for twenty-four hours. Make a list of the creations you will have the chef prepare for you, and describe what each will taste like.

What is the most memorable meal you have ever eaten? Describe the meal and the experience.

Cannabis beverages are the future. From non-alcoholic beers and wines to teas and seltzers, you can drink your way to high. Create a cannabis beverage of your own. Name it, and describe the flavors and experience of your drink.

Edible flowers are a fun way to garnish a dish or beverage. Imagine there is an edible cannabis flower. What does it taste like? What is the texture like? Describe how it feels when you eat it.

Edibles have come a long way—from OG weed brownies to unique offerings like infused-chocolate almonds, shrimp chips, and macaroons. What's the best edible you've ever had? Describe your high.

Make a list of your five ultimate junk foods, and why you love them. Do your cravings coincide with certain times of the day or month?

Open your fridge. With only the ingredients inside of it, write a new recipe and name it.

Fair and carnival food is uniquely famous for being fun, strange, deep-fried, and delicious. Countless options include deep-fried Oreos, pizza cones, cannoli dessert nachos, and deep-fried peanut butter and jelly sandwiches. Create your own fair-food offering. The more innovative, the better.

You're floating down a lazy, liquid-cheese river. The cheese is golden, and your raft is made from a soft salted pretzel. Continue the story of your experience on the lazy, cheese river.

What are some foods you disliked as a kid? What do you think of them now? How have your tastes changed as you've gotten older?

Do you consider yourself an adventurous eater? Why or why not?

Write a bucket list of ten places where you would love to eat. It could be street vendors, fine dining establishments, or your great-grandparents' kitchen.

You get a golden ticket to visit any candy factory in the world, real or imagined. What candy factory would you choose, and why? Describe what you hope to get out of your visit. Is it to get unlimited tastes of that candy? Is it to see how it's made?

What's a food you love and had in the past that you can no longer get? What do you remember about the taste and experience?

Commercial food collaborations are all the rage—think Cheetos Mac 'n Cheese, Pringles Scorchin' Hot Ones, Kit Kat Blueberry Muffin bars, and Taco Bell Doritos Locos Tacos. Create your own dream-food collaboration of brands, and write a story about its origins.

Deliciousness is in the air. It's peak summer, and you're a guest at an elaborate picnic. You smell barbecue and charcoal. Describe the table spread, meats, and sides, and don't forget about dessert!

You've chartered a private plane with enough fuel to get you anywhere in the world for dinner. Where do you ask your pilot to take you, and, once there, what do you order?

What's the craziest food you've ever eaten? Tell the story of how you ate it and the experience of its flavor, whether good, bad, or something in-between.

Describe your most magical high-food story. It could be a time when food tasted extraordinarily good, or a time you realized being high made food better.

Cannabis-infused pizza has popped up all over the country. Create your stoned pizzeria menu. Are the toppings traditional or innovative? Are there savory and sweet options?

Imagine it's a cold and rainy day; thunder echoes outside as you prepare soup. What kind of soup are you making? Is there a type of soup that gives you extra comfort? Be detailed.

Is a hot dog a sandwich? Why or why not?

You're out living in the wild, surviving off the land. It's a good thing that you know how to grow your own food. Describe in detail the gardens you've set up for yourself. What do you grow for food?

You turn a corner to discover the most vibrant and bustling street filled with food vendors. Describe in detail what you see, smell, and taste from three different food vendors.

Ice cream comes in so many flavors, textures, and types. Describe in detail the best ice cream you have ever had and the experience, including where you were and who you were with.

Let's talk breakfast. Eggs and bacon? French toast with powdered sugar? Cold pizza? Describe your perfect breakfast and what it means to you.

If you had to pass on one favorite recipe to the next generation, what would it be? Would you put your own spin on it?

You've invented a cannabis-infused energy bar. How does it fuel your body? What ingredients does it contain? And what does it taste like?

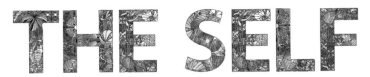

THE SELF

You've ventured to outer space, into nature, and through all the deliciousness that is food. Now I'll ask you to turn inward as we journey into the forest of *you*. Cannabis heightens consciousness, so it can be a great tool for introspection. It allows us to go beyond our ego into our most authentic selves. So take advantage of this opportunity. You are one-of-a-kind; your experiences are your own; and you are a well of inspiration waiting to be tapped into. Some great strains for this section are: Northern Lights, Hawaiian Haze, and Super Suver Haze. Let your mind wander as you honor and acknowledge your highest self.

Speak to your inner child. Pick any age (before you were eighteen) and write your younger self a letter.

Write about an activity you love doing while high and why you love it. It could be cleaning your house, meditating, or hiking. Anything goes!

Write down ten things you are grateful for in this moment.

Plan a "Treat Yourself" day. Imagine you've got unlimited funds and can go anywhere. Anything is possible in this reality. The only requirement is that the plan is about *you* only. Where do you go? What do you do? Do you explore? Do nothing? Make your plan below.

How did you discover cannabis? Write your cannabis origin story.

Describe yourself with the first twenty words that come to mind.

Write a short love or thank-you letter to cannabis. You could thank it for great memories or deep relaxation. What would you tell the plant if it could speak your language?

Compose a bucket list of ten things you want to do in the future. They could be goals, dreams, or everyday wishes.

Let's do a cannabis free-word association: Using one of the following words, write the first thing that comes to mind. It could be a story, poetry, a list, or utter nonsense. Here are the words: Blue Dream, Kush, joints, stoned, bong hit.

Describe the best day you've ever had.

List twenty things that make you happy. They could be big things or small things. The only requirement is that they spark joy.

_____

_____

_____

_____

_____

_____

_____

_____

_____

_____

_____

_____

_____

_____

_____

_____

You can time-travel into the future. What time period do you choose, and why do you go there?

If you could have a superpower, which one would you choose, and why? How would you use it?

Write a short paragraph about the highest high you ever experienced. It could be a literal high or a high in life.

What are your top-five simple pleasures?
These are the little things that bring you
contentment.

Write down a few sentences about a recurring dream you've had, or a theme that comes up often. What do you suppose this dream or theme is telling you?

Write about the present moment. Take in the details: smells, sights, sounds, and textures. Just observe, being fully present, and write down what you notice.

Write about a person, fictional or real, who inspires you. Explain the impact they've had on you and how they've inspired you.

Free write for three minutes about your favorite movie, book, or song.

_____

_____

_____

_____

_____

_____

_____

_____

_____

_____

_____

_____

_____

_____

_____

_____

You're building a time capsule to be opened in 150 years. What objects from the present do you put in it? Why did you choose these objects?

Complete this prompt: I love getting
high and . . .

Write about the differences in your personality and perspective while high versus while sober. What strengths come with each for you?

Describe your best "highdea" (an idea you had while high). It could be brilliant, strange, revolutionary, or silly.

You've been chosen to star in a reality TV show, real or imagined. What reality show do you become the star of and what's its premise?

If there was one thing you could manifest in the future, what would it be, and why?

What's something you have never tried
(a place, activity, hobby, etc.) but have always
wanted to explore? What's one, tiny step you
could take to come closer to doing it?

What color do you believe represents your personality? Why do you relate to this color?

Write yourself a quick thank-you note for something you have overcome, changed, or achieved. It could be as simple as drinking a glass of water every morning or as complex as tackling a major life challenge.

What are you feeling right now? Write a brain dump of all your emotions.

What is the most surprising thing you have learned thus far in your life?

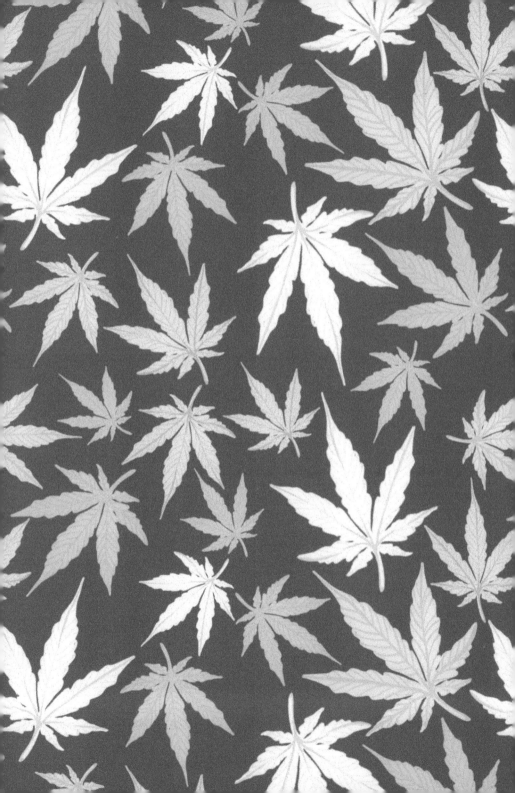

THE PAST

A lot happened before we came on the scene. Countless civilizations, people, and events have led up to where we are today. The past—both historically and personally—can serve as an important guide to the present and future, as well as a great tool for unlocking new ideas. While you can't go back in time, you can learn from and explore the past creatively. My favorite strains for this section are Amnesia Haze, Space Queen, and Chemdog.

If you could go back in time to have lunch with one person in history, who would it be and why? Write three questions you'd like to ask them.

Cannabis has historically defined many different time periods, from the 1920s jazz scene to the 1960s and beyond. If you could time-travel to any period in cannabis history, what era would you go back to, and why? What would you most want to experience?

What was your first memory?

In five sentences, tell the history of planet Earth from the perspective of the sun.

Cannabis use dates back to 2800 BCE, when it was recorded as a Chinese medicine. Write a few sentences about how you've used cannabis as medicine in your journey.

If you could change one thing about the past, what would it be, and why?

It's the New York City blackout; the year is 1977. You're walking down the street when the lights go out. Do you go home, or do you journey into the darkness? What happens? How do you feel?

Hemp, the low-THC version of cannabis, has historically been used to make many items, including clothing, paper sails, and rope. You're now tasked with designing something with hemp fiber. What would you create, and why?

You've just arrived home to find a visitor from ancient Greece, who is staying with you for the next twenty-four hours. It's your job to show them the modern world. Plan the next day with your ancient friend. Be as detailed as possible. What will you show them, and why?

When you were growing up, what did you think a "good life" meant? How has it changed as you've gotten older?

What time period inspires you the most? Write a few sentences about your favorite parts. Be vivid in your descriptions.

You're heading out west for the California Gold Rush of 1849. Where do you journey first? What are you hoping to accomplish?

You're allowed a visit from ten people from one time period. Who are your visitors, and which time period are they from?

You're sitting on the beach when you see an ancient, glass bottle wash ashore. It's clearly been afloat for many years. Inside is a message. It reads . . .

Write an invented history of the joint.

You're granted the chance to revisit a single day in your past. What day do you choose, and why?

You're sitting on the coastline when a Viking ship appears. What happens next?

If you could talk to ancient humans about our evolution, what would you ask them? What would they say?

You're the first person on Earth to ever get high. Describe this discovery and what you do with it.

You've traveled to a time when cannabis is largely underground, and you're in charge of your own cannabis speakeasy. Describe the people, the decor, and its most famous patron.

It's 1963. You're on Hippie Hill in San Francisco, lounging on a blanket with friends. The sun begins to set, and your friends spark up a joint. Free write for three minutes continuing this story.

It's the 1930s, and you're in a jazz club in Harlem. Describe the night. Is it a peaceful evening watching jazz? Do you smoke cannabis with Billie Holiday?

In 1954, pot brownies were formally introduced to American consciousness, thanks to *The Alice B. Toklas Cookbook*. Make up your own story about the origins of the first pot brownie.

You've traveled back in time with the task of explaining social media to a stranger. What era do you visit, and what do you tell this stranger? How do they respond?

One day, we will all be part of history. Write a letter about the present to someone who will read it in the year 3000.

Who was your first friend? Are you still in touch? If not, what do you imagine they might be up to now?

You've entered the Museum of Your Past. What important artifacts are on display, and how would you describe them?

Think about a struggle or mistake you made in the past. What was it, and what did you learn from it?

If you had to live out the remainder of your days in another era, which period would you choose to live in, and how would you get by?

If you could go back in time and learn something about yourself sooner, what would it be, and how would it change things?

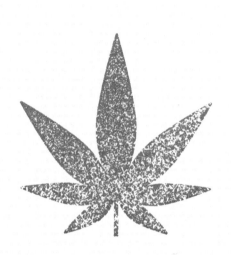

About the Author

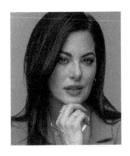

After more than fifteen years in the cannabis trenches, Kush Queen CEO and founder **Olivia Alexander** was determined to change the face of the cannabis business for the better. By focusing on CBD-infused products and continually improving formulas designed to work with the feminine body, Kush Queen has become one of the most respected cannabis-wellness brands on the market. The combination of its game-changing nanotechnology and advanced minor cannabinoid formulas, along with a fun, educational approach to cannabis, has earned Olivia the title "The Mariah Carey of Weed" by *Elle* magazine and the "Queen of CBD" by the *Los Angeles Times*. Olivia is the author of *The Essential Guide to Cannabis for Women* and has over one billion impressions as a social media influencer, sharing her own mental health and alternative medicine journey on Instagram and TikTok. She lives in Dana Point, California, with her two Samoyed children and life partner.

CPSIA information can be obtained
at www.ICGtesting.com
Printed in the USA
JSHW031521211122
33587JS00007B/57